T0144842

PADMA BASIC®

ANCIENT TIBETAN HERBAL FORMULA

NAN KATHRYN FUCHS, PH.D.

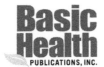

Basic Health
PUBLICATIONS, INC.

The information contained in this book is based upon the research and personal and professional experiences of the author. It is not intended as a substitute for consulting with your physician or other healthcare provider. Any attempt to diagnose and treat an illness should be done under the direction of a healthcare professional.

The publisher does not advocate the use of any particular healthcare protocol but believes the information in this book should be available to the public. The publisher and author are not responsible for any adverse effects or consequences resulting from the use of the suggestions, preparations, or procedures discussed in this book. Should the reader have any questions concerning the appropriateness of any procedures or preparation mentioned, the author and the publisher strongly suggest consulting a professional healthcare advisor.

Series Cover Designer: Mike Stromberg
Editor: Carol Rosenberg
Typesetter: Gary A. Rosenberg

Basic Health Guides are published by
Basic Health Publications,
Inc.www.basichealthpub.com

ISBN: 978-1-59120-113-7 (Pbk.)
ISBN: 978-1-68162-766-3 (Hardcover)

Contents

Introduction to the Updated and Expanded Edition

In the 1960s, an ancient Tibetan herbal formula was introduced to Switzerland, carried thousands of miles and preserved through multiple generations from its original Himalayan origins. Since its "discovery" by Swiss pharmaceutical scientist Karl Lutz, this formula, known in the United States as Padma Basic®, has been the subject of over fifty published clinical studies. In fact, this remarkable preparation remains one of the most widely researched herbal formulas in the world. As the impressive body of scientific evidence about Padma Basic expands, its reputation as a powerful and versatile therapy continues to grow as well. Today, this unique combination of twenty-one natural ingredients is widely regarded as a safe and effective remedy, useful for some of our most critical health concerns including heart disease, chronic inflammation, and cancer.

When the original edition of this book was published in 2003, the information was enthusiastically received by patients and doctors of diverse backgrounds. From conventional medical practitioners to integrative physicians and health-conscious consumers, people were eager for substantial data on natural remedies. As a result, the number of health professionals recommending Padma Basic grew beyond traditional holistic practices. Integrative MDs, dentists, nurse practitioners, cardiologists, osteopaths, and many others began to discover Padma Basic's remarkable properties. Patients shared the research with their doctors, and more doctors began recommending Padma Basic to their patients.

This revised, updated edition of the original Padma book includes two new studies on the formula. One is a meta-analysis highlighting Padma Basic's benefits against intermittent claudication and peripheral arterial occlusive disease (PAOD). The other is a clinical study demonstrating Padma Basic's efficacy in addressing acute dental pulpitis and as a possible root canal alternative. Both of these studies add further weight to Padma Basic's extensive resume of published clinical data.

In fact, as peer-reviewed research on Padma Basic continues, this unique formula may be regarded as a significant icon, symbolizing the advancement of integrative medicine today. With its impressive credentials and widespread use, Padma Basic represents the bridging of East and West; the scientific substantiation of ancient botanical wisdom; and the strategic application of herbs and nutrients that offer remarkable healing benefits. Most notably, an essential principle of integrative medicine is clearly reflected in Padma Basic's formulation: a synergistic blend of powerful yet gentle ingredients that fight disease and simultaneously support health from multiple angles.

In the years to come, I hope to see this dynamic integration of science and tradition gain even greater momentum, as leading research continues to advance our understanding of nature's most powerful healers.

—*Nan Kathryn Fuchs, PhD*

A History of Tibetan Medicine

More than two thousand years ago, high in the Himalayas, Tibetan medicine was born. It evolved out of the recognition of a strong connection between man and nature, and its remedies were made from local herbs, spices, and native plants. Tibetan doctors developed herbal formulas over the centuries, carefully documenting the most effective blends for future generations. Fortunately, part of each doctor's training was to memorize these ancient texts, for when the Chinese invaded Tibet in 1950 and most medical textbooks and doctors were destroyed, many of these formulas survived. Padma Basic is one of them. Used for the past fifty years in the treatment of cardiovascular disease, immune enhancement, multiple sclerosis, asthma, chronic infection, cancer, and more, Padma Basic is the most well known of all Tibetan herbal formulas.

Tibetan medicine is based on the principle that health is achieved through balance in all areas of our lives. We should not be too sad or too happy, too carefree or too worried, too warm or too cold. In keeping with these principles, Padma Basic is a powerful antioxidant formula that helps restore balance in part by cooling the body internally. Many of the ingredients in Padma Basic increase circulation and reduce inflammation, while also regulating immunity. For this reason it is used extensively for heat-related conditions, poor circulation, inflammation, and infections.

Padma Basic has been widely studied for circulatory disorders like peripheral artery disease, arteriosclerosis, and intermittent claudication. It also suppresses an overactive immune system and boosts low immunity, making it a powerful and safe immune regulator, useful for many autoimmune issues. As if this wasn't enough, research has found Padma Basic to be effective in the treatment of asthma, diabetes, multiple sclerosis, and cancer. Yet despite this impressive body of data, it looks like we have just begun to understand a fraction of Padma Basic's many applications.

Of all herbal combinations, Padma Basic appears to be one that is most ideally suited to diseases of the twenty-first century. These life-threatening conditions, such as heart disease, cancer, and type 2 diabetes, represent a class of illnesses termed "Western diseases" because they're commonly linked to imbalances in diet, lifestyle, and environmental factors. As a comprehensive Tibetan herbal formula, Padma Basic supports the treatment of these diseases because it functions on various levels to bring the body back into balance.

1

Understanding Tibetan Medicine

Tibetan medicine is one of many traditional medical systems around the world that is rooted in the concept of balance. When we are in balance we are healthy, while imbalances often lead to illness. This ancient practice of medicine is a complex system that reflects the close relationship between man and nature. At the very heart of Tibetan medicine are three subtle principles or bodily energies. These energies—wind, bile, and phlegm—have both physical and emotional properties.

Wind is associated with movement, including the circulation, digestion, and the nervous system. Bile relates to the metabolism and liver function, and phlegm is connected to anything that lubricates the body and the memory.

Within these three bodily energies are five elements: air, fire, water, earth, and ether. Each one, except ether, plays a role in the classification of illnesses that are considered hot, cold, or neutral. Too much heat or cold creates imbalance, and imbalance leads to disease. Inflammatory bowel disease is one example of excessive heat, while a sluggish digestion can be a sign of too much cold. An illness is often a result of an excess of either one or the other.

The three bodily energies affect the way we feel both physically and mentally, and we are healthy when there is harmony between them. Tibetan doctors believe that imbalances between these energies often originate from three emotional excesses. The first one is greed, or a continuous craving for power and material possessions. The second emotional excess is envy or anger toward people who have more than we do. The third, ignorance, is based on a refusal to see things as they are and to accept them. So an important aspect of Tibetan medicine consists of recognizing these excesses and bringing our thoughts and desires into balance. Another is recognizing the role of proper diet on our health.

The foundation of Tibetan medicine is based on the balance between the three bodily energies and the five elements they contain. Treatment consists of more than the bed rest and symptom-suppressing medications we associate with Western medicine. It begins with behavior modifications—changing the attitudes that shape our actions—and then implementing the appropriate dietary changes that can help restore us to balance. Herbs follow, along with other physical therapies, which may include massage, mineral baths, acupuncture or acupressure, laying-on of hands, visualization techniques, and meditation.

Tibetan medicine relies heavily on herbal remedies that either have a cooling or warming effect. These formulas are designed to address the cause of the problem and restore balance to the three bodily energies. Of all aspects of Tibetan medicine, herbal remedies are the most easily accessible to individuals throughout the world and the most easily assimilated into any lifestyle. You don't need a doctor skilled in Tibetan medicine to benefit from thousands of years of accumulated knowledge. Although this system of healing is sophisticated and complex, you can begin to use it by understanding which remedy is appropriate for you, locating a good quality formula, and using it regularly over a period of time.

Fortunately, it's not necessary to choose between Western medicine and Tibetan medicine. Each has its place in our health and healing and each can complement the other. In Europe, Canada, and the United States, Tibetan formulas are now frequently taken along with pharmaceuticals.

Tibetan herbal remedies are particularly useful in chronic conditions since they are designed to address the underlying cause of an illness, not just mask its symptoms. These formulas tend to work slowly and steadily to rebalance the body, while Western medications give faster results by suppressing uncomfortable symptoms. Results from herbs are not usually seen overnight, but when they do occur they are often profound and lasting. Because they work on such a deep level, eliminating the cause for a disease at its core, it is important to be patient and persistent when using herbal remedies.

The plants and minerals used in these ancient formulas have particular pharmacological properties that correspond to the five elements, helping to restore balance. In addition, when the ingredients are blended in specific combinations and quantities they create a new substance that has even greater healing abilities. This is an example of *synergy*, where the total effect is greater than the sum of each of its parts.

One of the most impressive of all Tibetan herbal formulas with strong research that supports its effectiveness is the cooling formula known as Padma 28 throughout Europe and Padma Basic in the United States. This ancient formula that originated in the Himalayas is now manufactured in Switzerland under strict quality-controlled conditions. Although some of its ingredients can only be found in parts of Asia, others come from herbs cultivated in Switzerland and from the world market for medicinal herbs.

At one time, the plants used in traditional Tibetan formulas were gathered high in the Himalayas near various villages and prepared by local doctors. As some of these doctors began to migrate to Siberia, Mongolia, and Europe due to the Communist occupation of China, they looked for other plants containing the same properties. Over the years, some of these formulas changed slightly, but their effectiveness continued. The current Padma Basic formula has been carefully evaluated and found to be accurate by Dr. Yeshi Donden, the Tibetan doctor who founded Tibet's premier medical school, *Men Tsi Khang*, and who was formerly the Dalai Lama's personal physician. The story of how this formula traveled from Tibet to Siberia and on to the United States is a fascinating one. Even more interesting is its wide variety of uses.

2

The Discovery
of Padma Basic

Padma Basic is one of many classic herbal formulas that originated in Tibet and was hand-carried through Mongolia to Siberia by followers of Tibetan Buddhism and Tibetan medicine during the Communist invasion. In the mid-nineteenth century, Alexander Badmajew, a Tibetan doctor who had left Tibet for sanctuary in Siberia, relocated to St. Petersburg and brought with him a suitcase stuffed with his precious collection of herbal formulas. They had become an integral part of his medical practice and he could not be without them. Among these formulas was one called Padma 28, the twenty-eighth formula in his collection. This formula is now also known as Padma Basic.

Other members of his family shared Alexander's passion for Tibetan medicine and used many of its traditional herbal formulas. His nephew, Vladimir Badmajew, became a well-known doctor in Poland who continued the family tradition of combining Tibetan and Western medicine to successfully treat his patients. And Vladimir's son, a surgeon named Peter, held on tightly to his family's inheritance of herbal formulas until a single event occurred that would introduce Padma Basic to the world.

This incident occurred in 1954 when a young Swiss pharmaceutical salesman, Karl Lutz, who was interested in Tibetan herbal remedies, attended a lecture on Tibetan medicine given by a Benedictine monk—Father Cyrill of Korvin-Krasinski. Karl was fascinated by Father Cyrill's talk and over the next ten years he studied the concepts, philosophy, and practice of Tibetan medicine by night while selling conventional pharmaceuticals by day. He kept in contact with Father Cyrill, pressing him for more information—far more than the Benedictine monk had. But what Father Cyrill didn't know, Peter Badmajew—whose father was the last traditional Tibetan doctor in the family's lineage—did.

Years before, Alexander Badmajew had tried to give the greatest gift in his possession—his family's treasured herbal formulas—to the Polish government in appreciation for giving him sanctuary in Poland. But the Polish government refused—not realizing the potential for their commercial use. The formulas remained in the Badmajew family where they were eventually passed along to Peter. And they might still be waiting for their value to be recognized if it was not for Karl Lutz's curiosity.

The more Karl learned about Tibetan medicine, the more he wanted to know. Father Cyrill introduced Karl to Vladimir Badmajew's widow, and through her he met Vladimir's son, Peter. Karl and Peter began to correspond, and Karl eventually invited Peter to visit him in Switzerland. The surgeon arrived with his family's herbal formulas tucked into his baggage, and the two men began to explore ways they could bring these Tibetan treasures to the Western medical community.

Karl had a wonderful idea. He was working for a Swiss pharmaceutical company. Surely they would want to manufacture and distribute such powerful formulas. Karl was so convinced of their great value that he sent them to the main office of his company, explaining his findings. To his surprise, the pharmaceutical company wasn't interested in them at all. What's more, they began to question Karl's loyalty. How could he possibly sell traditional pharmaceutical drugs when he was so interested in herbs and their folklore? Eventually, they gave him an ultimatum. Karl could remain with the pharmaceutical company selling conventional medicines, or he could leave his job and devote his life to Tibetan medicine.

This decision was not an easy one; Karl was married with three small children to support. But he knew in his heart that the herbal formulas from the Badmajew family would be lost forever without his help, and he was so convinced of their value that he left his secure position to work with Peter.

By combining their knowledge of pharmaceuticals with the preparation and use of these ancient remedies, the two men realized it might be possible to produce a few of the formulas. Coincidentally, at this time a group of Swiss doctors who were members of the Swiss Study Group of Tibetan Medicine were finding that some of these same formulas were particularly effective with their patients. These physicians helped Karl document a precise list of the indications for fourteen of these traditional herbal formulas so they could be registered as medicines. Of all the formulas Peter had inherited, Padma 28, now known as Padma Basic, one of the primary longevity formulas in all Tibetan medicine, seemed to have the widest number of applications.

Karl struggled with this project for twenty years and founded Padma, Inc., the Swiss company that still manufactures Padma Basic along with a number of other Tibetan herbal formulas. To this day, Padma, Inc. is the only Western company in the world that manufactures Tibetan herbal formulas. The remedies they produce all meet international pharmaceutical standards of purity. By refusing to give up his dream, Karl was able to bring Padma Basic to the world of natural medicine.

The Formula

Padma Basic is a cooling formula that is particularly effective in supporting circulation and reducing inflammation. It consists of nineteen different plants along with camphor and calcium sulfate. These ingredients are rich in antioxidants and contain polyphenols like bioflavonoids and tannins, as well as other potent phytonutrients (plant chemicals). The antioxidants promote good circulation and a healthy heart, and the combination of ingredients reduces inflammation and supports the immune system, making Padma Basic an excellent formula for general health and longevity. But it does much more.

Pharmaceuticals frequently have one or two activities while plants tend to have many. This is why it is not as easy to pigeonhole the properties of an herbal formula as easily as a drug. The dozens of nutrients and chemicals contained in plants often regulate, rather than increase or decrease, an action. When they help regulate body functions they are called adaptogens, because they help the body adapt whether it's "turned up" or "turned down." This means that if your immune system is suppressed, adaptogenic herbs will support and strengthen it. If your immune system is overactive and you have an autoimmune disease, the same herbs will reduce its hypersensitive response. Many of the herbs in Padma Basic have adaptogenic qualities.

The primary functions of the herbs used in Padma Basic include reducing inflammation and increasing circulation. But some of these plants also work specifically on the lungs, making this formula valuable for respiratory illnesses. Each plant within the formula has specific medicinal qualities, but it is not these individual qualities that are responsible for the formula's success. When the plants are blended together or combined, they create a remedy that is stronger and more effective than is each of its ingredients alone.

Padma Basic is made from finely ground raw particles of plant materials that are put into capsules. Each batch is tested for quality and purity using the latest state-of-the-art technology. Before any herb is processed, it is tested for pesticides, heavy metals, bacteria, and mold. Only pure ingredients are used. The quantity of each herb is carefully measured using sophisticated testing called "chemical fingerprinting." This guarantees that the formula contains the precise quantity of tannins, flavonoids, and other ingredients needed to get the desired results.

The plants used in Padma Basic are Iceland moss, costus root, neem fruit, cardamom fruit, red saunders, chebulic myrobalan, allspice fruit, bael tree fruit, columbine, English plantain, licorice root, knotweed, golden cinquefoil, clove flower bud, resurrection lily rhizome, heart-leaved sida, valerian root, wild lettuce leaf, and calendula flower. A chart giving the botanical and common names for every herb, along with some of its properties and the quantity used in this formula, can be found in the Appendix.

The formula we know today as Padma Basic began as Padma 28. The two formulas are nearly identical. The only difference is that Padma 28 contains a minute quantity of aconite, an ingredient that is not permitted in herbal formulas sold in the United States. Nevertheless, the action of the two formulas appears to be identical. Padma 28 is still sold in Europe, but North American countries import Padma Basic. To avoid confusion, the name Padma Basic is used throughout this book.

Each of the ingredients in Padma Basic has at least one of the following actions:

1. Contributes to the primary effect, such as increasing circulation or reducing inflammation.

2. Supports the primary effect.

3. Counteracts any negative side effects from any other ingredients. Western medicines often have side effects that are normally addressed by taking other medications, but traditional Tibetan formulas contain within themselves the qualities needed to counterbalance any side effects.

3

Padma Basic and Healthy Circulation

Your circulatory system carries blood throughout your body through your veins and arteries, nourishing your tissues with oxygen and nutrients. Poor circulation reduces the ability for the food and oxygen you need to reach your cells. A healthy diet and regular exercise can help support good circulation, while smoking, a poor diet, and inactivity can lead to a buildup of plaque resulting in blockages in your veins and arteries. They can also contribute to circulatory problems that affect your legs and heart. Preventing these blockages is not only a key to staying healthy; it's an important factor in looking and feeling young. Blockages cause arteries to become narrow and stiff, reducing circulation. The result is that when less oxygen and nutrients are supplied to waiting cells, you feel tired and run down.

For optimal circulatory health, you need to prevent the buildup of plaque in your arteries, and studies show that Padma Basic is particularly effective in keeping veins and arteries free from plaque. While surgery and chelation therapy are two modern methods of reversing atherosclerotic plaque, Padma Basic has been found to be effective both in helping to prevent and treat this buildup at a fraction of the cost and with no side effects.

Supporting good circulation is vital in slowing down the aging process and increasing longevity. This is why many doctors today are using this herbal formula in their antiaging nutritional programs.

Peripheral Artery Disease and Intermittent Claudication

Atherosclerotic plaque that builds up in the legs is called peripheral artery disease or peripheral vascular disease. When leg pain develops intermittently from this buildup of plaque the condition is called intermittent claudication. Intermittent claudication is a widespread problem that affects 12 percent of all adults over the age of fifty and limits their ability to get the exercise they need for a healthy heart and weight control. Both peripheral artery disease and intermittent claudication are complications of atherosclerosis.

When we're sitting down, our blood vessels carry two cups of blood a minute to our legs. But when we're exercising, the body's need for oxygen increases and the quantity of blood that's needed jumps to three or four quarts of blood every minute. Arteries that have become obstructed with plaque just can't carry enough blood or oxygen to our legs. The result is muscle pain that begins after even mild exercise— like walking one or two blocks—and disappears with complete rest. Current studies indicate that Padma Basic is well suited to both peripheral artery disease and intermittent claudication, although its notoriety occurred quite by accident when it was used to resolve a difficult case of intermittent claudication.

In the mid-1960s, a Swiss medical doctor, Dr. Charles, had a high-profile patient who suffered from intense leg pain. His patient was the municipal president of a neighboring town who was in such pain from advanced obstructions in the arteries of his legs that he was barely able to walk. Dr. Charles had tried every medication he could think of for his patient, but nothing helped. Then he remembered being given a Tibetan herbal formula by a pharmaceutical salesman, Karl Lutz. The salesman had told the doctor that this formula was effective in relieving leg pain. With no other options open for him to try, Dr. Charles gave his patient the herbal formula. To his surprise and delight, it worked beautifully. After taking the Padma Basic formula for a number of weeks, his patient was able to walk a considerable distance without any pain.

Dr. Charles was delighted to find an answer for his patient, but could this success be duplicated? He was anxious to know, so he tried the formula on several of his patients with atherosclerosis. Their conditions improved as well. Word spread about Dr. Charles's success, and more and more doctors began to use Padma Basic. The formula was then used in double-blind, placebo-controlled studies at the Zurich University Clinic and eventually throughout the world.

There are currently more studies using Padma Basic for peripheral artery disease and intermittent claudication than there are for a buildup of plaque in the arteries of the heart. This is because it's both quicker and easier to test the arteries in the legs. However, the principle is the same. If Padma Basic can reduce the buildup of plaque in arteries in the legs, it stands to reason that it is also removing the buildup of plaque in coronary arteries.

Research on Padma Basic and Reduced Leg Pain

The results of a randomized double-blinded study published in the medical journal *Angiology* in 1993 looked at thirty-six patients with an average age of sixty-seven who suffered from intermittent leg pain for five years. Each patient was given either a placebo or two capsules of the Padma Basic formula twice a day for four months. At the conclusion of the study, the patients who took Padma Basic were able to walk twice as far as before without leg pain, while those who took the placebo had no improvement.

In another study conducted in Germany and published in 1985, patients with intermittent leg pain who took the herbal formula for only one month had a similar 100 percent increase in the distance that they could walk without pain. Clearly, this herbal formula not only works well—it has the ability to work quickly.

Just how does Padma Basic prevent this buildup of plaque? A Polish study published in 1991 suggests it affects high-density lipoprotein (HDL) and low-density lipoprotein (LDL) cholesterol. Padma Basic appears to increase the helpful cholesterol (HDL) and reduce the harmful cholesterol (LDL). HDL is the slick form of cholesterol, while LDL is sticky. When you have enough HDL, it keeps the sticky fats from adhering to the arterial walls. On the other hand, if you have too much LDL, these fats can cause a buildup of plaque that often leads to poor circulation and leg pain. Here's what the 1991 study found:

Fifty patients who had arteriosclerosis and intermittent claudication were given Padma Basic or a placebo for four months. At the end of this study, the patients taking the herbal formula were able to walk further without pain than those who took the placebo, just like the participants in previous studies. But these researchers did more than look at pain versus no pain. They examined blood lipid levels (fatty acids and cholesterol) in all of the participants as well and found that the herbal formula had additional benefits. It reduced cholesterol and triglyceride (a harmful fat) levels. It also lowered LDL cholesterol, reducing the stickiness that can lead to more plaque buildup. Just like the previous studies, the patients who took the placebo had no change in their pain or in lipid levels.

In 2006, a meta-analysis review of Padma Basic's clinical data in the treatment of intermittent claudication was published in the journal *Atherosclerosis*. Six controlled clinical studies have analyzed the effects of Padma Basic on peripheral arterial occlusive disease (PAOD) on 444 patients. This review examined five of the six studies; review authors also obtained original data from the authors of the published research and reports, as well as from the manufacturer. The meta-analysis showed Padma Basic to be significantly effective in relieving symptoms of PAOD. A number of subjects experienced reduced leg pain and were able to increase walking distance by over 100 meters. The authors conclude that the effects of Padma Basic are comparable to standard PAOD medications.

When we look at Padma Basic's antioxidant activity in the following chapter, we will see another way in which the formula affects LDL. Not all LDL is harmful—as some people think. We need some LDL to help transport vitamins E and A through our bloodstream. But when LDL oxidizes it becomes harmful. Too much cholesterol, or too few antioxidants, causes LDL to oxidize. Many of the herbs in Padma Basic have antioxidant activity.

Smoking and Atherosclerosis

Smokers are prone to atherosclerosis because nicotine promotes blood clots. It does this by increasing fibrinogen (a blood protein) in the blood. The more fibrinogen you have, the more easily blood will clot. These blood clots, along with decreased circulation, lead to pain in the legs that is often referred to as "smokers' leg."

Your body's wisdom can be seen in its many checks and balances. You don't want your blood to be too thick or too thin. If it's too thick it can lead to blood clots. On the other hand, if your blood doesn't clot well, a minor cut could cause a great loss of blood. To keep your blood from getting too thin, your body makes substances that keep it thick enough. A Danish researcher at the University of Copenhagen, Dr. Kaj Winther, found that Padma Basic neutralizes the substances that thicken blood, allowing blood clots to dissolve more quickly.

Coronary Artery Disease and Angina

When atherosclerotic plaque builds up in the coronary arteries, it is called atherosclerosis or arteriosclerosis—hardening of the arteries. The arteries, which originally are flexible, become stiff and hard. Blockages caused by plaque leave little room for blood to travel through them, and this slows down the circulation. When circulation is reduced, less oxygen can be pumped through the blood and into waiting tissues. Both exercise and eating heavy meals can cause the heart to pump faster than usual. At these times, the blocked arteries are unable to carry enough oxygen to the heart, causing pain. This condition is known as angina pectoris. Angina pain is not an indication of a heart attack, but rather a signal of insufficient oxygen.

Padma Basic is effective against angina pain. In one study, a group of fifty patients with angina were given a placebo for two weeks followed by two weeks of taking the Padma Basic formula. The dose was two capsules two times a day. The severity and frequency of their angina attacks were compared, along with their response to therapy, ability to exercise without pain, ergonomic tests, and platelet aggregation (the ability of their blood to clot). A significant decrease in angina attacks was observed in 69 percent of subjects. Treatment with Padma Basic resulted in decreased heart rate, systolic blood pressure, and platelet aggregation.

The effect on lipids was examined in another animal study. In this one, a group of researchers studied the effect of Padma Basic on rabbits given a high-fat diet. One group of rabbits ate a high-fat diet alone for three months while another group ate the same high-fat diet plus Padma Basic. Blood lipid levels fell dramatically and insulin levels became normal in the rabbits that were given Padma Basic.

This study did more than just look at Padma Basic's effect on lipids. It also measured atherosclerotic plaque. The rabbits on the high-fat diet alone had an average increase in plaque of over 67 percent in just three months. The rabbits that ate the same diet and received Padma Basic had an increase of only 15.5 percent. Padma Basic may not completely stop the formation of plaque in arteries, but even with a poor diet that is high in fats, it slows down its progression.

The best way to avoid a buildup of plaque and all forms of heart disease is through a healthy diet, regular exercise, and not smoking. This is often easier said than done. Many people who lead busy lives and eat on the run don't fully realize that their lifestyle is contributing to the beginnings of a chronic illness—until it's too late. Other people are too busy to stop and re-evaluate their lives, and make the necessary lifestyle changes that could contribute to their health. The new field of antiaging medicine works in part by interrupting a silent, slow progression toward disease and reversing it through nutrient therapy. Padma Basic seems to be ideally suited as an important supplement for either the prevention or treatment of one of the greatest health problems of modern times: heart disease. Obviously, no supplement holds the complete answer to a serious chronic condition like atherosclerosis, but it appears that Padma Basic is an important addition to a comprehensive healthy heart program.

Atherosclerosis means more than a buildup of plaque and a narrowing of arteries. We're now learning that it is also an inflammatory process triggered by oxidative stress and the presence of harmful free radicals. Padma Basic works by reducing both plaque and inflammation. Inflammation is a major underlying factor in a number of chronic illnesses, and this is discussed in more detail in the following chapter. But it is important to understand now that the cooling properties of the herbs in Padma Basic make it an ideal formula for all inflammatory processes, including atherosclerosis.

4

Padma Basic and Inflammation

An inflammation is like a fire in your body. It creates heat and spreads if you don't put it out. Left alone, an inflammation may lie smoldering, burning slowly and undetected without you ever knowing it's there. Eventually, it can lead to chronic illnesses, but not all inflammation is harmful. Acute inflammation can actually be beneficial. It protects you by helping your body burn up foreign materials like toxins and bacteria, preventing them from spreading and causing damage to tissues and organs. The heat, pain, redness, and swelling from inflammation are all protective responses that help your body eliminate foreign substances and prepare injured tissues for repair.

Chronic inflammation is damaging. When tissues become inflamed repeatedly or consistently they break down faster than they can be repaired. This process leads to numerous diseases over time. It can take decades before a minor inflammation develops into diabetes, cancer, or heart disease, but chronic inflammation rarely just "goes away." As we said earlier, inflammation has recently been found to be a major risk factor for heart disease and is directly associated with a buildup of plaque in the arteries. But it's also a component of every condition that ends in "itis" (arthritis, dermatitis, gingivitis, hepatitis, colitis, pancreatitis, and so forth); some forms of cancer; asthma; and inflammatory bowel disease.

As common as it is, the association between inflammation and chronic illness has been overlooked because it's often so difficult to detect. Now we're finding it is at the core of dozens of diseases. If you have any minor condition associated with inflammation, like swollen gums (gingivitis), you may have a low-level chronic inflammation that's just waiting to become a more serious problem. By taking safe anti-inflammatory substances like those found in foods and herbs, you are gently encouraging your body to return to a state of balance . . . and health.

Fire Starters and Fire Fighters

Some substances increase inflammation and others put out its fires. To reduce chronic inflammation you first need to reduce your exposure to anything that promotes and feeds it. This means reducing two kinds of dietary fats (omega-6 fatty acids and trans-fatty acids), refined sugar and grains, and free radicals.

Omega-6 fats are commonly found in vegetable oils including corn, soy, safflower, peanut, and cottonseed. Replace them with heart-healthy olive oil whenever possible. Trans-fatty acids are found in partially hydrogenated vegetable oils. You'll find them in many salad dressings, nondairy creamers, margarines, and baked goods. Read labels carefully and choose foods without hydrogenated or partially hydrogenated oils. In some cases, eliminating foods with harmful oils will also reduce your intake of sugar.

Nothing feeds inflammation like refined sugar, white flour products, and foods that turn into sugar quickly (known as high-glycemic foods). Replace refined sugars with whole grains and fruits whenever possible.

A diet high in fresh fruits and vegetables also reduces inflammation in two ways. First, these foods cool the body just like the herbs in Padma Basic. Second, they're also high in antioxidants. Without sufficient antioxidants you run the risk of having too many free radicals and more inflammation.

Free Radicals, Oxysterols, and Inflammation

Free radicals are molecules that damage cells and speed up the aging process. They contribute to coronary artery disease and cancer, two diseases associated with aging. There's no way to escape free radicals. They're found in sunlight, air pollutants, cigarette smoke, and prescription drugs, and are even produced by your white blood cells to destroy unwanted bacteria and viruses. If you have enough antioxidants in your diet and supplements, you can keep these harmful free radicals in check. Otherwise, they can run rampant and damage molecules in their paths. When fats in your body are attacked by free radicals they become rancid. This rancidity is called *lipid peroxidation,* a process associated with the beginnings of atherosclerosis and cancer.

Free radicals stimulate inflammation. They not only help white blood cells stick to damaged cells and microbes the body needs to eliminate, they also stick to normal cells. When they do, this can lead to blockages in joints and arteries. Iron is a heavy metal that contributes to the production of free radicals. Research has shown that one of Padma Basic's antioxidant properties is its ability to grab onto iron molecules and remove them. Iron is a pro-oxidant, a metal that contributes to oxidation and has been known to contribute to diseases.

Free radicals also make oxysterols, a harmful, oxidized form of cholesterol that causes plaque to form on artery walls. In fact, it is not high cholesterol, or even LDL (harmful) cholesterol, that contributes to heart disease. LDL cholesterol becomes harmful when it oxidizes into oxysterols. To control inflammation, you need to reduce both oxysterols and high amounts of free radicals. Ordinarily, free radicals are kept in check by antioxidants, chemicals that protect cells from damage caused by oxidation. But in today's polluted world, you may not have enough antioxidants in your diet to protect yourself adequately from rancid fats and oxysterols.

Reducing free radicals has an additional benefit. It slows down the aging process by keeping you healthy and free from chronic debilitating illnesses. When excessive free radicals are destroyed as quickly as they're produced, your body stays young from the inside out and you are less likely to have oxidative, stress-related diseases like asthma, cancer, and arteriosclerosis. Free radicals can be kept under control with various antioxidants like vitamins E, A, and C, found in a healthy diet high in fresh fruits and vegetables. But these same antioxidants are found in herbs as well, like many of the herbs in Padma Basic. A study on cell cultures published in the journal *Inflammopharmacology* found that Padma Basic blocked cells from being attacked by oxidants and other destructive substances.

The herbs in this Tibetan formula contain tannins and flavonoids, powerful antioxidants called polyphenols that protect plants from fungus, ultraviolet radiation, and other environmental toxins. Polyphenols also protect us from damage caused by free radicals. Enzymes made in our bodies neutralize some free radicals, but enzymes alone may not be enough to handle all the free radicals produced in today's toxic world.

Antioxidants Affect All Inflammation

When you cool down an inflammation in one area in your body, you put out fires in other areas. This explains why your dermatitis may clear up when your inflammatory bowel disease is treated with anti-inflammatory drugs. Similarly, the cooling properties in the antioxidants in Padma Basic work on all inflammatory processes simultaneously. As one inflammation subsides, so do others.

We don't yet know how or why the antioxidants in particular plants work the way they do since pharmaceutical companies are reluctant to fund studies that investigate the effects of substances they can't patent. So the pharmacology of each herb used in Padma Basic is not completely understood at this time. We do know, however, that many of the herbs in this formula have known anti-inflammatory properties. For instance, cloves (*Syzgium aromaticum*) contain oil that prevents arachidonic acid, the fat found in animal products, from becoming rancid, and rancid fats lead to the production of free radicals. Licorice root (*Glycyrrhiza glabra*) is another herb that is well known for its anti-oxidant properties.

As more and more studies are conducted with this formula it is becoming clear that the antioxidant and anti-inflammatory properties of Padma Basic come not only from the individual substances, but also from the interactions that occur when they are combined.

Nitric oxide is a tiny molecule that's found throughout the body. While no one really knows what it does, too much nitric oxide appears to be at the core of many illnesses. For instance, nitric oxide appears to be high wherever there is inflammation. Padma Basic has been found to prevent the production of nitric oxide. One study on mouse macrophages found that several herbs contained in Padma Basic blocked the production of nitric oxide. This may be one explanation for its effectiveness as an anti-inflammatory formula.

5

Padma Basic and the Immune System

Y_ou are as healthy as your immune system is strong. A healthy immune system protects your body from harmful viruses, bacteria, parasites, molds, dead cells, and allergic responses to undigested food. A strong immune system will protect you from the minor discomforts of colds or flu as well as from devastating conditions like cancer and autoimmune diseases. A weak immune system, on the other hand, makes you vulnerable to pathogens that contribute to disease. So your immune system is your key to staying healthy, vital, and young. Padma Basic appears to work on both minor and major immune problems by acting as an immune regulator. It turns on an underactive immune system and turns down one that is overactive.

Supporting the Immune System

Perhaps there is no illness that is as strongly associated with the immune system as cancer. When your immune system is strong, renegade cancer cells can be identified and destroyed just like other substances your body identifies as foreign invaders. But when your immune system is weak, these cancer cells produce an enzyme that helps them attach to blood vessels. Then they can break through these blood vessels and travel to other organs. The process where cancer spreads to other locations is called metastasis. All cancers become more dangerous when cancer cells travel to other sites and the cancer spreads like wildfire.

Many of us begin life by having a strong immune system. As we age, however, the immune system changes and produces fewer protective T cells. (T cells are white blood cells that target and destroy viruses, tumors, and microbes that cause infections.) This means that as we get older our immune system tends to become weaker. Fortunately, we can strengthen it at any age. The immune-supporting activity of Padma Basic, added to its other properties, increases its effectiveness and value in the treatment or prevention of numerous chronic illnesses.

For instance, an animal study was conducted that examined the effects of Padma Basic on the immune reactions in rabbits with atherosclerosis. Researchers noted a significant reduction in the size of atherosclerotic plaques in the aortas of rabbits given Padma Basic. In addition, the formula restored the rabbits' immune function. The researchers believe that there is a connection between atherosclerosis and the immune system that explains Padma Basic's beneficial effects of boosting the immune system and reducing arterial plaque.

Antibacterial Activity

In addition to viruses and tumors, pathogenic, or harmful, bacteria affect your immune system. Once again, it's all about balance. Your body contains hundreds of strains of both helpful and harmful bacteria. Harmful bacteria are kept from multiplying out of control when you have sufficient healthy bacteria. Taking supplements of friendly bacteria like *acidophilus* and *Bifidobacteria* can help restore the balance of good to bad bacteria. Antibacterial substances found in many herbs also keep harmful bacteria under control.

Some harmful bacteria like *Streptococcus* and *Listeria* can cause minor problems like eczema and sore throats. Or they can cause more serious conditions like scarlet fever, food poisoning, or meningitis. One research study compared Padma Basic with five European herbs known to have antimicrobial activity. These herbs had been used topically with success against mild skin infections and eczema. All of the individual herbs as well as the Padma Basic formula exhibited evident antibacterial effects against Gram-positive bacteria *in vitro,* including methicillin-resistant *Staphylococcus aureus* (MRSA) and *Listeria monocytogenes.*

Chronic Dental Pulpitis

In 2006, a clinical study on Padma Basic was published in the international medical journal, *Forsh Komplementarmed.* The study showed the herbal formula's antibacterial and anti-inflammatory effects for chronic dental pulpitis and its use as a possible alternative to root canal treatment. Dental pulpitis is usually caused by cavities that degrade the tooth enamel and dentin, allowing bacteria to infect the tooth pulp. While bacterial infection is usually the culprit, sometimes trauma from repeated dental work or other injuries can be the cause. Symptoms of chronic dental pulpitis include radiating pain, throbbing pressure, and tooth sensitivity (though some cases don't show any symptoms until it's too late).

In this study, forty-nine pulpitis patients took two capsules of Padma Basic, twice a day, for fifteen days. Fifty-five percent (twenty-seven patients) were completely free of pain within one month—some within a few days. Eighteen percent (nine patients) were gradually pain free within two months. Eight percent (four patients) had a slower recovery, and 18 percent (nine patients) had to undergo root canal or extraction in spite of taking Padma Basic. Altogether, over 80 percent of the patients experienced complete remission, and most of the patients remained symptom free for more than three years. No side effects were reported. The success of Padma Basic in treating chronic dental pulpitis can be attributed to its powerful immune-boosting, anti-inflammatory, and antibacterial properties.

Many of the foods and herbs we eat have antibacterial properties. Of the two, herbs usually have stronger antibacterial properties than foods. Rosemary, garlic, and oregano are examples of culinary herbs with antibacterial properties, and they can be included in your daily diet for a healthy immune boost. But the amount of herbs we use in cooking is rarely enough to reduce high quantities of pathogenic bacteria. This is why a concentrated herbal formula will always outperform individual culinary herbs.

Antiviral Activity

A strong immune system inactivates viruses, so the presence of a chronic virus can be a sign or warning of a suppressed immune system. Some viruses, like herpes simplex, become active when the immune system is suppressed due to stress. In this way, herpes can be an early warning that your immune system needs support.

While herpes can be uncomfortable, hepatitis can be deadly. Hepatitis is an inflammation in the liver that is usually caused by one of a number of hepatitis viruses. However, other viruses, bacteria, and reactions to drugs or alcohol can also trigger it. The inflammation caused by hepatitis damages liver cells and in some cases can lead to death. The best way to control hepatitis is to inactivate it. This normalizes liver enzymes, reduces inflammation, boosts the immune system, and prevents liver damage.

Hepatitis is difficult to treat. Conventional treatment often consists of expensive medications that either don't work or have serious side effects. One of these is interferon, a pharmaceutical drug used to treat hepatitis C. Interferon works by increasing antiviral activity and decreasing white blood cells. The result appears to block the replication of the hepatitis virus by preventing vulnerable cells from being infected.

Numerous studies using the Padma Basic formula have found it to be effective against the hepatitis B virus. Current clinical experience indicates that it is equally effective in treating hepatitis C. In clinical and experimental studies on the herpes virus published in Germany, Padma Basic was found to significantly increase the body's production of interferon and regulate the immune system.

A study published in *Phytotherapy Research* in 1993 followed thirty-four patients with chronic hepatitis and treated them with Padma Basic for one year. They were monitored both clinically and with a variety of laboratory tests. At the end of the year, more than 75 percent of the participants either had normal T-cell counts or had a stronger immune system. At the same time, there was no liver inflammation.

A larger study followed 126 adults and 52 children with chronic hepatitis B over a period of two years. They were each given two capsules of Padma Basic three times a day. At the end of the study, 15 percent of the patients had no viral activity. Ninety percent of them had an improvement in their T-cells and had a marked improvement in their overall immune response.

6

Padma Basic
and the Lungs

Allergies and bacterial infections can lead to more serious lung problems like bronchitis, pneumonia, and asthma. Just as many herbs contain antioxidants and anti-inflammatory substances, they also tend to have antimicrobial activity. The herbs in Padma Basic have all of these properties, making it particularly well suited for lung problems in both adults and children. The studies on its effectiveness for respiratory infections in children are further evidence of its safety and efficacy.

Bronchitis, Pneumonia, and Respiratory Infections in Children

Children with compromised immune systems come down with frequent colds that often lead to bronchitis, pneumonia, or bacterial lung infections. These children often grow into adults with chronic lung problems and suppressed immune systems. The traditional treatment for these lung problems is to give children course after course of antibiotics. The antibiotics work until the child either builds up immunity to the drug, or the bacteria or virus mutates into a form that the antibiotics can't recognize. Then that particular antibiotic is no longer effective and the search goes on for other drugs that can do the job . . . at least for a while.

Meanwhile, an inflammatory process or bacterial infection is left to cause damage to young lung tissues. The future health of a child is influenced by the amount of antibiotics they take at a young age and the number of years they have been exposed to processes that damage tissues. We've seen that Padma Basic is effective against *Streptococcus* and *Listeria* in cell cultures, but what effect does this Tibetan formula have on people with bacterial infections? And if it works on adults, is it safe and effective to give to young children?

It not only works well, but studies show that it is safe. A three-year study followed 300 children with lung problems. Each child had at least one lung infection a month for the preceding nine months, including bouts of bronchitis or pneumonia for at least three of those months. All steroids were discontinued three months before they were given Padma Basic. Two weeks before beginning Padma Basic, all antibiotics were stopped. The children were then given the herbal formula for a period of nine months. At the end of the study, more than 70 percent of the children had improved. In many of them, their T-cell count had normalized. No side effects were reported.

In another study, a group of researchers followed nineteen children between the ages of two and four who had bronchitis or pneumonia at least once a month for the past nine months. They were caught in a cycle of infections, antibiotics, and more infections. All of the children were taken off antibiotics for the duration of the study. They were given one capsule of Padma Basic three times a day for one month, followed by two weeks without the herbal formula. Then they were given the same dose for another two weeks.

Their blood was examined twice during the study for serum bactericidal activity (SBA); SBA is a substance that protects against infections. The blood was also tested against three strains of bacteria: one strain of *Salmonella* and two strains of *E. coli*. Children taking the Padma Basic formula had an increase of protective SBA in their blood and at least a twofold decrease in pathogenic bacteria. There was no change in SBA levels in the control group. So, Padma Basic increased an infection-fighting substance in the blood and was effective against some strains of the *Salmonella* and *E. coli* bacteria associated with food poisoning.

E. *coli* is the bacterium that was found in some beef products several years ago that caused food poisoning. Some children became sick and a few of them died. Padma Basic could offer protection from foodborne illnesses caused by *Salmonella* and *E. coli* in children, older adults, and people with compromised immune systems.

Other studies on recurring respiratory infections in children showed that Padma Basic corrected and regulated their immune systems and reduced the frequency and severity of infections. Benefits continued even after children stopped taking the formula. A study of sixty-one children with recurrent respiratory infections found an 80.4 percent decrease in the frequency of infections even after Padma Basic had been discontinued for a period of nine months. Instead of using antibiotics, parents might want to consider using Padma Basic for lung problems in their children. And adults who have frequent colds, flu, and bronchitis may find it effective in stopping their cycles of illness.

Asthma

There appears to be a strong link between allergic rhinitis, commonly known as allergies, and asthma. The common denominator is the presence of inflammation in nasal, sinus, and bronchial passages. Allergies often precede asthma. In fact, 10 percent of all Americans suffer from seasonal allergies—twice as many as in 1970. From 19 to 38 percent of all people with allergies in the United States progress to asthma, and the increased inflammation from rhinitis adds to this risk.

Specific immunotherapy is widely used for allergies, and we know that Padma Basic helps regulate the immune system. In addition, since this herbal formula is effective against inflammatory conditions, and both allergic rhinitis and asthma are inflammatory diseases, it stands to reason that Padma Basic would be an effective adjunct in the prevention and treatment of both asthma and allergies.

7

Padma Basic and Cancer

Many factors contribute to the complex category of diseases we know as cancer. This is why there is no one solution. Researcher and oncologist Daniel Clark, MD, councils doctors to "detoxify and support the immune system." This is good advice for any chronic illness, but it is perhaps even more appropriate in the case of cancer, a disease associated with cell aging.

This aging is not necessarily a result of a person's biological age, but often a condition where the immune system is unable to function properly. A healthy immune system can destroy and eliminate damaged or renegade cells and remove pathogenic bacteria and viruses. A toxic, overloaded, and weakened immune system allows diseased cells to multiply and form into tumors. Certainly, a key to both the prevention and treatment of any cancer is to strengthen the immune system and remove excessive toxins.

You may remember that free radicals are molecules that damage cells and contribute to inflammation. Chronic inflammation further damages cells, creating a cycle that is difficult to break. Damaged cells usually contain an antigen that helps the killer cells in your immune system recognize them as foreign bodies that need to be destroyed. But some cancer cells are clever enough to remove or cover up this antigen, allowing them to elude the killer cells and stick more effectively to one another. When cancer cells cluster together and adhere to one another they create tumors.

One way to prevent or reduce your risk of cancer is to reduce your number of damaged cells. Reducing oxidative stress can do this. Radiation and chemicals like those used in chemotherapy increase oxidative stress, leaving cancer patients more vulnerable to an even weaker immune system. This is why some doctors are now using Padma Basic along with chemotherapy and radiation treatments for their cancer patients. The herbal formula, high in antioxidants, reduces some of the damaging oxidants created by chemotherapy and radiation. A combination approach using Padma Basic along with traditional cancer treatments can allow the chemotherapy and radiation to destroy cancer cells with less residual damage.

Several studies have shown Padma Basic's effectiveness in reducing cancers both in cell cultures and in human clinical trials. A laboratory study using leukemia cells found that Padma Basic inhibited the growth of these cancer cells and accelerated their death. The Tibetan herbal formula appeared to make the cancer cells more sensitive to destruction.

It is more important to stop cancer cells from spreading to other sites than to kill these cells in a cancerous tumor. Tumors can be removed and often prevented from growing. But cells from a primary tumor, called daughter cells, can break off from the tumor and travel through the bloodstream. If they're not recognized by the immune system and destroyed, they will attach themselves to blood vessels in an attempt to break through to get to other organs. This process of spreading is called metastasis and metastasis can be lethal, especially when the immune system is compromised.

At the Hadassah University Hospital near Jerusalem, Dr. Israel Vlodavsky studied Padma Basic in women with breast cancer. He found that Padma Basic blocked the formation of the enzyme that helps cancer cells stick to blood vessels. By blocking this enzyme, Padma Basic kept breast cancer from spreading. We know that Padma Basic strengthens the immune system. This combination of supporting immunity and preventing metastasis makes Padma Basic a valuable adjunct in the prevention and treatment of cancers.

8

The Future
of Padma Basic

We know from a number of clinical and laboratory studies that Padma Basic has powerful activities against intermittent claudication and inflammation. Each study using this ancient formula points to a number of additional applications for which it appears to be extremely helpful. Here are a few of them.

Autoimmune Diseases

Autoimmune diseases like lupus, psoriasis, Crohn's disease, rheumatoid arthritis, and multiple sclerosis are all conditions where the immune system attacks its own tissues. Viral and bacterial infections, stress, and genetics may all contribute to these diseases, and preliminary studies indicate that Padma Basic may be effective in their treatment as well.

Rheumatoid arthritis in children responds to Padma Basic's ability to regulate an overactive immune system. In a six-month clinical study, nineteen children with juvenile rheumatoid arthritis (JRA) were divided into two groups. One group was given two to four capsules of Padma Basic daily for six weeks; the other group received thymus extract suppositories for four weeks. JRA patients experienced improvements using both formulations, including a reduction of symptoms and improved laboratory tests. In addition, neither formulation had any side effects. The researchers of this study suggest that

Padma Basic may be used as an alternative to orthodox medical treatment for rheumatoid arthritis.

Multiple sclerosis (MS) is a progressive neurological disease, primarily affecting women, caused by an autoimmune attack on the central nervous system. Spontaneous remissions may occur, but the disease frequently progresses until the patient is wheelchair-bound and unable to control bodily functions.

In the early 1990s, researchers studied 100 people with chronic progressive multiple sclerosis and gave half of them two capsules of Padma Basic three times a day for one year. The control group was given nothing. Only their symptoms were treated. At the end of the study, 44 percent of the patients on Padma Basic had a general improvement. They had increased muscle strength and either a decrease or disappearance of any disorders affecting their sphincter muscles. None of the control group felt any better, and 40 percent of them deteriorated. If Padma Basic can stop or slow the progression of MS, it may be a valuable addition to a treatment program.

Vascular Alzheimer's Disease

Alzheimer's disease is the most common form of senile dementia. It affects 10 percent of people over sixty-five and nearly half of the population over the age of eighty-five. It is characterized by a buildup of plaque on nerve endings that causes nerves connecting segments of the brain to die. A lack of blood to the brain caused by constricted arteries is thought to be a vascular form of Alzheimer's. It may be closely associated with coronary artery disease because more than 85 percent of people with coronary artery disease have been found to have plaque in their brain tissues that looks just like the plaque found in people with Alzheimer's disease. What's more, when these people had coronary artery surgery, the plaque in their brain tissues cleared up.

There were marked improvements in a small observational study using Padma Basic on older adults with Alzheimer's disease conducted in the mid-1980s. Thirty-four people were given one gram of Padma Basic a day in divided doses for six months (equivalent to one capsule three times a day). At the end of the study, the majority of patients had significant improvements in their memory, mental alertness, energy, attitude, and general well-being. As we saw earlier in the studies on peripheral artery disease, Padma Basic reduces arterial and vascular plaque. This appears to be the mechanism responsible for the improvement in people with a vascular form of Alzheimer's disease. Future double-blinded studies are needed, but the application in treating and preventing Alzheimer's looks promising.

Cell damage caused by oxidation also contributes to Alzheimer's disease. The antioxidants in Padma Basic provide a second line of defense in preventing and slowing down the progression of this condition.

Alcoholism

Padma Basic won't cure alcoholism, but in at least one study it protected the liver against damage from alcohol in laboratory animals. Prolonged use of alcohol raised liver enzymes, cholesterol, and triglycerides in rats. When the rats were given the Padma Basic formula in addition to alcohol, there was a significant reduction in liver enzymes and lipids. It stands to reason that this formula would help normalize liver function in recovering alcoholics and would protect people from liver damage caused by weekend drinking binges.

Sports and Exercise

Whether you are a professional athlete or a weekend warrior, the repeated physical strain from participating in various sports can lead to tendonitis (tennis elbow), sprained ankles, sore muscles, and stress on joints. Traditional treatment consists of anti-inflammatory medications and increasing circulation to the affected site. This is precisely what Padma Basic does.

Gabriele Feyerer, in her book *Padma* (Lotus Press, 2003) reports that two Moroccan ultramarathon runners, the Ahansal brothers, who run and won the *Marathon des Sables* (running more than 145 miles in six days) and the Swiss Alpine Marathon numerous times, found they recovered faster, had fewer leg cramps, and less inflammation after taking Padma Basic. They've been using this Tibetan formula for years. Other athletes have found similar effects. It would make sense for high school athletes, professional athletes, and people who have strenuous exercise sessions to take these herbs after heavy workouts.

Padma Basic doesn't increase an athlete's performance directly, but it does speed up the recovery time. The dosage for athletes depends on the intensity of the training, but the recommended amount varies from two to six capsules a day in divided doses.

Ulcers

Duodenal ulcers heal slowly because irritating enzymes and other substances are constantly traveling through the small intestines where the duodenum is located. To interrupt the inflammation caused by this irritation and allow ulcers to heal, researchers gave Padma Basic to twenty-three patients with peptic duodenal ulcers. At the end of their month-long study, nearly half of the patients who took Padma Basic had improved.

Diabetes-related Illnesses

We're just beginning to understand the role for Padma Basic in the treatment of diabetes. Diabetes frequently occurs in people with circulatory problems, and many diabetics who have normal LDL cholesterol levels progress to coronary heart disease (CHD) and strokes. The two conditions appear to be interrelated.

The group of drugs called statins may reduce a diabetic's risk for CHD. A recent study by the Heart Protection Study Collaborative

Group found that when statins were given for five years to diabetics with no sign of CHD, fewer major vascular events occurred. One of the side effects from taking statins, however, is that they reduce the levels of coenzyme Q_{10} (CoQ_{10}) in brain and heart tissues. Seventy-five percent of patients with heart disease have low levels of CoQ_{10} compared with healthy people.

The idea is to reduce the risk for vascular problems without lowering the amount of nutrients essential to good heart health. This is another application for the use of Padma Basic. Its antioxidants can contribute to increased circulation and reduced buildup of plaque.

Gabriele Feyerer reports a case of a woman with diabetes who had a leg wound so severe that her doctor was considering amputation. An open wound on her toe had refused to heal and her circulation was becoming more and more impaired. After taking Padma Basic for several months, her circulation improved and the wound began to heal. Seven months after starting the herbal formula, to her doctor's surprise, the healing was complete.

9

How to Use
Padma Basic

Padma Basic is not a "magic bullet." Think of it instead as a major ingredient in a comprehensive program including a healthy diet, supplementation, and regular exercise to support and restore your health. A full daily dose of Padma Basic is two capsules taken three times a day, but this amount may be too much to begin with, and two capsules twice a day may be sufficient for some people depending on their weight and the severity of their health problems. It may also be more than necessary for less serious and less chronic conditions. Here are some general guidelines.

For chronic conditions:

• Begin taking one capsule two times a day for three days

• Increase to two capsules two times a day for three days

• Increase to two capsules three times a day for 2 to 24 months, depending on the condition and its severity

For hepatitis, multiple sclerosis, and immune dysfunction:

• Follow the dosage directions above

• Continue at full dosage for a longer period than 24 months as directed by a qualified integrative doctor.

For circulatory problems:

• Begin with two capsules three times a day for two to four months

- Reduce to two capsules two times a day for a total of six months

Maintenance dose:

- One capsule two times a day

For children:

- One capsule three times a day

Ideally, Padma Basic should be taken half an hour before, or two hours after meals with a full glass of water. There are no known interactions between this herbal formula and any medications. However, if you are taking any homeopathic remedies or prescription drugs it is best, when possible, to leave a gap of one and a half to two hours between taking any other formulations/medications and Padma Basic.

Conclusion

Few herbal formulas have been as rigorously tested as Padma Basic for safety, efficacy, or mechanisms of action. Though we are certainly seeing progress in integrative and complementary medical research, more work needs to be done.

As you have seen, Padma Basic already has many applications based on extensive scientific research. It reduces inflammation, increases circulation, decreases atherosclerotic plaque, and regulates the immune system. It also helps the body fight bacterial and viral infections.

Nearly 150 Swiss doctors have been using Padma for decades and have observed numerous other conditions where it has been effective. These include memory problems, tinnitus, visual problems, back and joint pain, dizziness, and fatigue. It is just a matter of time before preliminary clinical observations are translated into further clinical trials and we find even more uses for this ancient herbal formula.

How can one formula be used successfully for so many different kinds of health problems? One answer lies in its adaptogenic qualities. Laboratory and clinical studies indicate that Padma Basic helps regulate the body. For instance, it supports an underactive immune system and turns down an overactive one.

Another answer is that the cooling qualities of the herbs in Padma Basic reduce all forms of chronic inflammation, and we are finding that ongoing inflammation is at the root of many health problems.

Of course, no one herb or herbal formula is the complete answer to any chronic health problem, and neither is Padma Basic. However, it does excel as an important addition to both conventional and integrative medicine. Clearly, Padma has so many beneficial qualities that it would be wise to incorporate it into a daily supplement regimen, especially for everyone over the age of forty.

Contents of Padma Basic

Scientific Name	Common Name•	mg per capsule	Fiber, Pectins	Essential Oils	Tannins	Amaroids	Flavonoids (Color)
Cetraria islandica	Iceland Moss	40	•			•	
Saussurea costus	Costus root	40	•	•	•		
Azadirachta indica	Neem fruit	35		•		•	
Elettaria cardamomum	Cardamom fruit	30	•	•			
Pterocarpus santalinus	Red saunders	30		•			•
Terminalia chebula	Chebulic myrobalan	30			•		
Pimenta dioica	Allspice fruit	25		•			
Aegle marmelos	Bael tree fruit	20	•		•		
Calcium sulfate	Gypsum	20					
Aquilegia vulgaris	Columbine herb	15	•		•		
Plantago lanceolate	English plantain herb	15	•		•		
Glycyrrhiza glabra	Licorice root	15	•				
Polygonum aviculare	Knotweed herb	15	•		•		•
Potentilla aurea	Golden cinquefoil herb	15			•		•
Syzygium aromaticum	Clove flower bud	12		•			
Kaempteria galanga	Resurrection Lily rhizome	10	•	•			
Sida cordifolia	Heart-leaf sida herb	10	•				
Valeriana officinalis	Valerian root	10		•			
Lactuca sativa	Wild lettuce leaf	6	•				
Calendula officinalis	Calendula flower	5		•			•
Cinnamomum camphora	Camphor	4		•			

•Standardized common names as given in *Herbs of Commerce*, American Herbal Products Association 2000.

Resources

**Producer of Padma Products
and Information about Padma**
Padma, Inc.
Unterfeldstrasse 1
CH-8340 Hinwil
Switzerland
Phone: +41 (0)43 343 44 44
Email: mail@padma.ch
www.padma.ch

**Padma Distributor
Europe/Netherlands**
SanoPharm Nederland bv
Prins Hendrikweg 2
3771 AK Barneveld
Phone: 0342-42-0714
Email: info@sanopharm.com

Padma Distributor Canada
Promedics
2498 W. 41st Ave.
Vancouver, BC V6M 2A7
Phone: 604-261-5057
Email: info@promedics.ca
www.promedics.ca

Padma Distributor U.S.
EcoNugenics, Inc.
396 Tesconi Court
Santa Rosa, CA. 95401
Phone: (800) 308-5518
Email: sales@econugenics.com
www.econugenics.com

**Information about integrating
ancient medicinal systems with
standard medical treatment**
www.dreliaz.org
Better Health Publishing
1007B West College Ave.
Santa Rosa, CA 95401
Phone: (707) 583-8619
Email: info@dreliaz.org

**Information about Tibetan
Medicine**
www.amfoundation.org/tibetan
medicine.htm

References

Bernacka, K., et al. 1991. "PADMA 28 and thymus extract on clinical and laboratory parameters of children with juvenile chronic arthritis." *International Journal of Immunotherapy* 7(3):143–147.

Bommeli, C., et al. 2001. "Clinical experiences in the general practice with a multicompound preparation derived from Tibetan medicine." *Erfahrungsheikunde* 50(11):745–756.

Brzosko, W. J., et al. 1986. "PADMA 28 in the treatment of chronic active hepatitis." *Biologische Medizin* 15(6):300–305.

Brzosko, W. J., et al. 1992. "Padma 28 in patients with chronic hepatitis B: clinical and immunological effects." *Schweiz Zschr für Ganzheits Medizin* 7(8; Suppl. 1):13–14.

Drabaek, H., et al. 1993. "A botanical compound, Padma 28, increases walking distance in stable intermittent claudication." *Angiology* 44(11):863–7.

Feyerer, G. 2003. *Padma: Integrating ancient wisdom and modern research using traditional Tibetan herbs for today's diseases.* Twin Lakes, WI: Lotus Press.

Fullemann, F. 2006. "Padma 28 in the treatment of chronic dental pulpitis: an observational case study in 49 patients." *Forsch Komplementmed* 13(Suppl. 1):28–30.

Gieldanowski, J., et al. 1992. "Padma 28 modifies immunological functions in experimental atherosclerosis in rabbits." *Archivum Immunologiae et Therapiae Experimentalis* 40(5–6):291–295.

Ginsburg, I., et al. 1999. "PADMA-28, a traditional Tibetan herbal preparation inhibits the respiratory burst in human neutrophils, the killing of epithelial cells by mixtures of oxidants and pro-inflammatory agonists and peroxidation of lipids." *Inflammopharmacology* 7(1):47–62.

Gladysz, A., et al. 1993. "Influence of Padma 28 on patients with chronic active hepatitis type B." *Phytotherapy Research* 7:244–247.

Hasik, J., et al. 1992. "Effectiveness of duodenal ulcer disease treatment by PADMA 28 and Padma 137." *Nowiny Lekarskie* (Poland) 2:40–44.

Heart Protection Study Collaborative Group. 2003. "MRC/BHF heart protection study of cholesterol-lowering with simvastatin in 5963 people with diabetes: a randomized placebo-controlled trial." *Lancet* 361(9374):2005–2016.

Jankowski, A., et al. 1986. "Treatment with PADMA 28 of children with recurrent infections of the respiratory tract." *Therapiewoche Schweiz* 2(1):25–32.

Jankowski, A., et al. 1991. "Influence of PADMA 28 on the spontaneous bactericidal activity of blood serum in children suffering from recurrent infections of the respiratory tract." *Phytotherapy Research* 5:120–123.

Khalsa, D. S. 1998. "Integrated medicine and the prevention and reversal of memory loss." *Alternative Therapies* 4(6):39–40.

Koh, Y. Y. and C. K. Kim. 2003. "The development of asthma in patients with allergic rhinitis." *Current Opinion in Allergy & Clinical Immunology* 3(3):159–164.

Korwin-Piotrowska, T., et al. 1992. "Experience of PADMA 28 in multiple sclerosis." *Phytotherapy Research* 6:133–136.

Melzer, J., et al. 2006. "Treating intermittent claudication with Tibetan medicine Padma 28: Does it work?" *Atherosclerosis* 189(1):39–46.

Moeslinger T., R. Friedl, I. Volf, et al. 2000. "Inhibition of inducible nitric oxide synthesis by the herbal preparation Padma 28 in macrophage cell line." *Canadian Journal of Physiology and Pharmacology* 78:861–866.

Panjwani, H. K. and M. D. Priestley. 1986. "Clinical evaluation of PADMA 28 in treatment of senility and other geriatric circulatory disorders: A pilot study." Study report/personal communication. New Jersey: 1–15.

Samel, Gerti, *Tibetan Medicine,* Little, Brown & Company, Great Britain, 2001.

Saputo, L. and N. Faass. 2002. *Boosting immunity: Balancing your body's ecology for maximum health.* Novato, CA: New World Library.

Schrader, R., et al. 1985. "Effects of the Tibetan herbal preparation Padma 28 in intermittent claudication." *Schweizerische medizinische Wochenschrift* 115(22):752–756.

Smulski, H. S. 1991. "Treatment of chronic ischemia of the lower extremities with complex herbal preparation." *Annales Academiae Medicae Stetinensis* 37:191–192.

Suter, M. and C. Richter. 2000. "Anti- and pro-oxidative properties of PADMA 28, a Tibetan herbal formulation." *Redox Report* 5(1):17–22.

Ueberall, F., et al. 2002, October 20–25. "The Tibetan herbal remedy PADMA 28 fights tumor cell growth in cell culture." 28th meeting of the Federation of European Biochemical Societies. Istanbul, Turkey. Abstract Number 363.

Vanderhaeghe, L. R, and P. Bouic. 1999. *The immune system cure.* New York: Kensington Books.

Weseler, A., et al. 2002. "Comparative investigation of the antimicrobial activity of PADMA 28 and selected European herbal drugs." *Forsch Komplementarmed Klass Naturheilkd* 9:346–351.

Winther, K., et al. 1994. "PADMA-28, a botanical compound, decreases the oxidative burst response of monocytes and improves fibrinolysis in patients with stable intermittent claudication." *Fibrinolysis* 8(Suppl. 2):47–49.

Wojcicki, J. and L. Smaochowiec. 1986. "Controlled double-blind study of Padma 28 in angina pectoris." *Herba Polonica* 32:107–114.

Wojcicki, J., et al. 1988. "Effect of PADMA 28 on experimental hyperlipidaemia and atherosclerosis induced by high-fat diet in rabbits." *Phytotherapy Research* 2(3)119–123.

Wojcicki, J., et al. 1989. "Inhibition of ethanol-induced changes in rats by PADMA 28." *Acta Physiologica Polonica* 40(4):387–392.

Index

About the Author

Nan Kathryn Fuchs, Ph.D., is a nutritionist in private practice in Sebastopol, California, as well as a health educator. She is the author of a number of books, including *The Nutrition Detective, Overcoming the Legacy of Overeating, User's Guide to Calcium & Magnesium,* and *Modified Citrus Pectin (MCP): A Super Nutraceutical.* She is also editor of *Women's Health Letter,* a popular newsletter (www.womens healthletter.com).